THE ULTIMATE VEGAN SAUCES AND FILLINGS COOKBOOK

50 delicious recipes that will make you fall in love with vegan cuisine

Laura Mckinney

the reader will render any resulting actions solely under their purview. There are no scenarios in which the publisher or the original author of this work can be in any fashion deemed liable for any hardship or damages that may befall them after undertaking information described herein.

Additionally, the information in the following pages is intended only for informational purposes and should thus be thought of as universal. As befitting its nature, it is presented without assurance regarding its prolonged validity or interim quality. Trademarks that are mentioned are done without written consent and can in no way be considered an endorsement from the trademark holder.

Table of contents

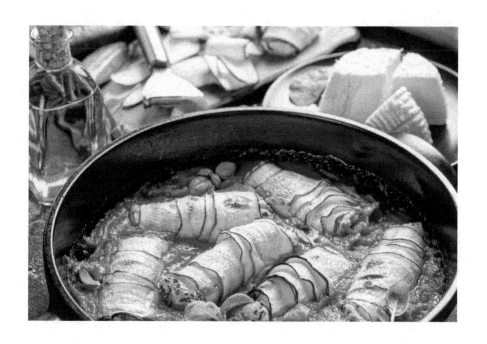

Introduction

Veganism is one of the most followed trends around the world today.

There are many people who have decided not to take more food products deriving from animal products and to follow a lifestyle in harmony with nature. The history of the vegan diet began in 1944 with a diet specially formulated for the purpose, five years later Leslie J Cross suggested the idea of veganism by supporting the idea of emancipating animals from human exploitation.

Over the years, veganism has become not only a food habit but a real lifestyle, influencing hundreds of thousands of people, for whom it shares an attitude of respect and protection of animals and nature in general.

Veganism involves the abolition of the diet of any food derived from meat, poultry, seafood, and dairy products. Contrary to what one might think, however, the vegan diet is very varied and full of succulent and very different dishes, to satisfy any preference. From breakfast to dinner you can vary to your liking with very good and satisfying sweet and savory dishes. The only condition is that each meal is made with ingredients of plant origin. And don't think that the vegan diet has limits on nutrients, because vitamins, minerals, and vital proteins can be taken from vegetables, fruits, cereals, nuts, and seeds. It will be enough to practice a little and the result will certainly be in line with our expectations, thanks also to an increasingly refined technology of cooking meals. Vegan food is very varied, from vegan ice cream, to burritos, cheese, burgers, mayonnaise and so much more. Being vegan does not mean depriving yourself of something, on the contrary, it means improving your lifestyle in harmony with the nature of which we are part.

The vegan diet also includes the consumption of lettuce, pasta, chips, bread, and various sauces.

The reasons that push people to become vague can be the most disparate, the lifestyle they assume certainly benefits everyone! The vegetable diet is sufficiently rich in iron, folic acid, magnesium, vitamins C and B1 which are essential for our body. At the same time, the vegan diet can never include a high amount of saturated fat and cholesterol.

Also, veganism has obvious health benefits, helping to prevent serious diseases such as stroke, type 2 diabetes, obesity, colon and prostate cancer, hypertension, and ischemic heart disease. There are no age preclusions to follow a vegan diet, however, we recommend greater attention to the daily meal ratio, to avoid nutritional deficiencies. __

In this cookbook, you will find 50 delicious recipes that will make you want to get up in the morning. There are recipes for every taste, just follow our advice and you can make real culinary masterpieces. Forget the boredom of thinking about what to eat, this cookbook will give you the right inspiration.

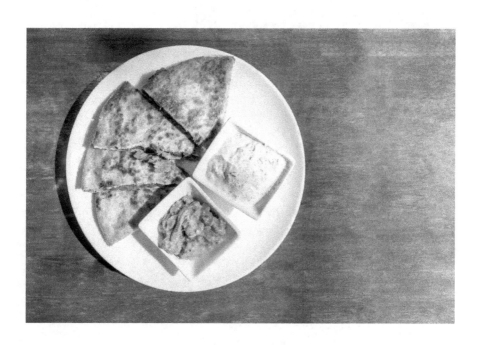

Vegan Gravy

Prep time: 10 minutes Cooking time: 15 minutes Servings: 4

Ingredients:

- ½ teaspoon cornstarch
- 1 cup almond milk
- 1 tablespoon olive oil
- 1 yellow onion, diced
- 1 cup mushrooms, chopped
- 1 teaspoon ground black pepper
- 1 teaspoon salt
- 1 teaspoon chili flakes
- 1 teaspoon oregano
- 1 teaspoon cilantro
- 1 teaspoon garlic, diced
- ¼ cup white wine
- ½ teaspoon miso paste
- 1 tablespoon soy sauce

Directions:

13. Preheat olive oil on Saute mode well.

14. Add diced onion, mushrooms, and garlic. Stir well and saute the vegetables for 5 minutes.

15.   After this, add ground black pepper, salt, chili flakes, oregano, cilantro, and soy sauce. Stir well.

16.   Add miso paste and white wine. Saute the mixture until it starts to boil.

17.   Then add almond milk and cornstarch. Mix it well.

18.   Close and seal the lid.

19.   Cook the gravy on manual mode (high pressure) for 2 minutes.

20.   Then make quick pressure release.

21.   Chill the cooked gravy little.

Nutrition value/serving: calories 203, fat 18, fiber 2.5, carbs 8.5, protein 2.7

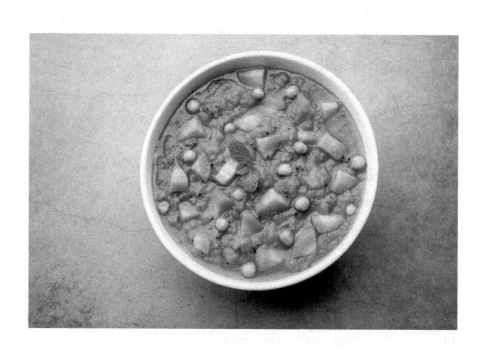

Samosa Filling

Prep time: 20 minutes Cooking time: 30 minutes Servings: 6

Ingredients:
- 1 cup chickpeas, soaked
- 3 cups of water
- 1 oz beetroot, chopped
- 1 garlic clove
- 1 tablespoon tahini paste
- 1 teaspoon salt
- ½ teaspoon harissa
- 2 tablespoons olive oil

Directions:
13. Place the soaked chickpeas and water in the instant pot.
14. Ad beetroot and garlic clove.
15. Close and seal the lid. Cook the ingredients for 30 minutes on manual mode (high pressure). After this, allow natural pressure release for 10 minutes.
16. Place 4 tablespoons of the liquid from cooked chickpeas in the blender.
17. Add cooked chickpeas, garlic clove, and beetroot.
18. Blend the mixture until smooth.

19.   Add tahini paste, salt, harissa, and olive oil. Blend the mixture well.

Nutrition value/serving: calories 180, fat 8.1, fiber 6.1, carbs 21.6, protein 7

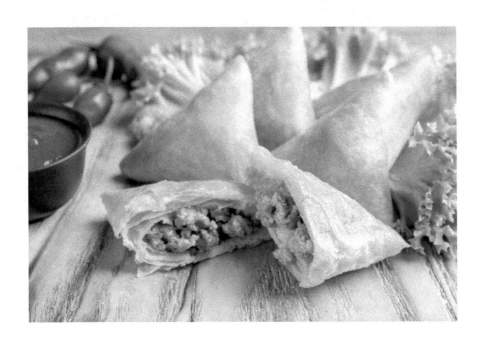

Cacao Spread

Prep time: 10 minutes Cooking time: 5 minutes Servings: 3

Ingredients:

- 1 tablespoon nuts
- ½ cup cashew milk
- 1 tablespoon raw cacao powder
- ¼ cup of sugar
- 1 teaspoon almond butter

Directions:

12. Blend together raw cacao powder and cashew milk.

13. Pour the liquid in the instant pot.

14. Add sugar and almond butter.

15. Cook the mixture on Saute mode for 5 minutes. Stir it from time to time.

16. Add nuts and mix up well.

17. Close the lid. Switch off the instant pot and let it rest for 10 minutes.

Nutrition value/serving: calories 142, fat 5.3, fiber 2.6, carbs 22.9, protein 2.5

Mexican Rice Filling

Prep time: 10 minutes Cooking time: 4 minutes Servings: 6

Ingredients:
- ½ cup black beans, canned
- 2 cups of water
- 1 cup fresh cilantro, chopped
- ½ cup corn kernels, frozen
- 1 cup of rice
- 1 teaspoon salt
- 1 tablespoon olive oil
- ½ teaspoon paprika
- 1 teaspoon chili flakes

Directions:
16. Place rice and water in the instant pot. Add salt and corn kernels.

17. Close and seal the lid. Set rice mode (high pressure) and cook rice for 4 minutes. Use quick pressure release.

18. Meanwhile, in the mixing bowl mix up together canned black beans, olive oil, paprika, chili flakes, and chopped cilantro. Mix up the mixture well.

19. When the rice and corn are cooked, chill them to the room temperature and add in the beans mixture. Mix up well.

Nutrition value/serving: calories 200, fat 2.9, fiber 3.4, carbs 37.4, protein 6.2

Cauliflower Sauce

Prep time: 10 minutes Cooking time: 10 minutes Servings: 3

Ingredients:
- 7 oz cauliflower
- 1 cup of water
- ½ cup almond milk
- 1 teaspoon salt
- 1 teaspoon ground black pepper
- 1 tablespoon wheat flour

Directions:
14. Place cauliflower and water in the instant pot.

15. Close and seal the lid. Cook the vegetable on Manual mode (high pressure) for 7 minutes.

16. Then make quick pressure release and open the lid.

17. Drain the water and mash cauliflower with the help of the fork

18. Add salt, ground black pepper, wheat flour, and almond milk.

19. Mix up the mixture well.

20. Cook it on Saute mode for 3 minutes more.

21. The cooked sauce shouldn't be smooth.

Nutrition value/serving: calories 120, fat 9.7, fiber 2.8, carbs 8.2, protein 2.6

Vegan French Sauce

Prep time: 10 minutes Cooking time: 6 minutes Servings: 5

Ingredients:

- 1 cup mushrooms, chopped
- ½ cup vegetable stock
- 1 teaspoon salt
- 4 oz firm tofu
- 1 tablespoon olive oil
- 1 teaspoon ground black pepper
- 1 tablespoon almond yogurt
- 1 teaspoon potato starch

Directions:

18.   Pour vegetable stock in the instant pot.

19.   Add mushrooms, salt, tofu, olive oil, ground black pepper, almond yogurt, and close the lid.

20.   Cook the dip on manual mode (high pressure) for 6 minutes.

21.   Then make quick pressure release.

22.   Open the lid and add potato starch.

23.   Blend the mixture with the help of the hand blender until smooth. The sauce is cooked.

Nutrition value/serving: calories 51, fat 4.3, fiber 0.5, carbs 2.4, protein 2.4

Pumpkin Butter

Prep time: 5 minutes Cooking time: 3 minutes Servings: 4

Ingredients:
- ½ cup pumpkin puree
- 3 tablespoons orange juice
- 1 tablespoon sugar
- 1 tablespoon almond butter
- ¾ teaspoon salt
- 1 teaspoon pumpkin pie spices

Directions:
14. Put pumpkin puree, orange juice, sugar, almond butter, and salt in the instant pot.
15. Sprinkle the mixture with pumpkin pie spices and stir well.
16. Close and seal the lid.
17. Cook the butter for 3 minutes on Manual mode (high pressure).
18. Then make quick pressure release. Open the lid and transfer the meal in the bowl.

19.   Chill it for 20-30 minutes before serving.

Nutrition value/serving: calories 53, fat 2.4, fiber 1.4, carbs 7.7, protein 1.3

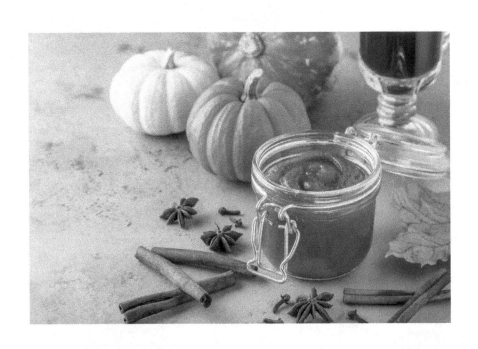

Cranberry Sauce

Prep time: 10 minutes Cooking time: 2 minutes Servings: 6

Ingredients:
- 8 oz cranberries
- 3 oz maple syrup
- 1 tablespoon lemon juice
- ¾ teaspoon dried oregano

Directions:
15. Place cranberries, maple syrup, lemon juice, and dried oregano in the instant pot. Stir gently.

16. Close and seal the lid.

17. Cook the sauce on manual mode for 2 minutes. When the time is over, allow natural pressure release for 5 minutes more.

18. Stir the sauce gently before serving.

Nutrition value/serving: calories 59, fat 0.1, fiber 1.5, carbs 13.1, protein 0

Spinach Dip

Prep time: 10 minutes Cooking time: 10 minutes Servings: 4

Ingredients:
- 1 teaspoon onion powder
- 2 cups spinach, chopped
- ½ cup artichoke hearts, canned, chopped
- 1 tablespoon olive oil
- 1 teaspoon ground black pepper
- 1 teaspoon salt
- ½ cup of coconut yogurt
- 1 teaspoon cornstarch
- 4 oz vegan Parmesan, grated

Directions:
15. Preheat the instant pot on Saute mode.
16. Then pour olive oil inside.
17. Add chopped spinach and chopped artichoke hearts.
18. Sprinkle the greens with ground black pepper and salt. Stir it well.
19. Close the lid and cook on Saute mode for 5 minutes.
20. After this, add coconut yogurt, onion powder, and cornstarch.

21.   Add grated Parmesan and mix up the mixture well.

22.   Cook it for 5 minutes more.

Nutrition value/serving: calories 150, fat 4.1, fiber 1.6, carbs 11.5, protein 13.3

Red Kidney Beans Sauce

Prep time: 10 minutes Cooking time: 35 minutes Servings: 4

Ingredients:
- ½ cup red kidney beans, soaked
- 2 cups of water
- 1 tablespoon tomato paste
- 1 bell pepper, chopped
- 1 teaspoon salt
- 1 teaspoon chili flakes
- ½ teaspoon white pepper
- 1 tablespoon corn flour
- ¼ cup fresh dill, chopped

Directions:
17. In the instant pot, combine together red kidney beans, water, tomato paste, chopped bell pepper, salt, chili flakes, white pepper, and dill.
18. Mix up the mixture well.
19. Close and seal the instant pot lid.
20. Set manual mode and cook the ingredients for 30 minutes.
21. Then use quick pressure release and open the lid.

22.   Add corn flour and mix up the sauce well.

23.   Close the lid.

24.   Saute the sauce for 5 minutes on Saute mode.

25.   Then stir it well and let chill till the room temperature.

Nutrition value/serving: calories 105, fat 0.6, fiber 4.7, carbs 20.4, protein 6.4

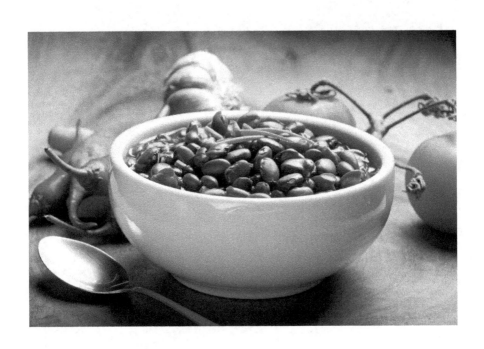

Cayenne Pepper Filling

Prep time: 5 minutes Cooking time: 15 minutes Servings: 2

Ingredients:

- 1 sweet potato, peeled, chopped
- 1 cayenne pepper, chopped
- ½ cup of water
- 1 tablespoon almond yogurt
- 1 teaspoon olive oil
- 1 carrot, grated
- 1 teaspoon mustard

Directions:

13.   Pour olive oil in the instant pot and preheat it on Saute mode.

14.   Add chopped sweet potato and cayenne pepper.

15.   Saute the vegetables for 5 minutes.

16.   Add grated carrot and stir it well.

17.   Then pour water in the instant pot and add mustard and almond yogurt. Mix up the mixture.

18.   Close and seal the lid.

19.   Cook the filling on Manual mode (high pressure) for 5 minutes. Then make a quick pressure release and transfer the meal in the serving plate.

Nutrition value/serving: calories 103, fat 3.2, fiber 3.5, carbs 17, protein 1.9

Vegan Cheese Sauce

Prep time: 10 minutes Cooking time: 6 minutes Servings: 4

Ingredients:

- 1 white potato, peeled, chopped
- 1 sweet potato, peeled, chopped
- 1 carrot, chopped
- ½ cup peanuts, chopped
- 1 tablespoon lime juice
- 1 teaspoon salt
- 1 teaspoon onion powder
- 1 teaspoon ground black pepper
- 1 teaspoon chili flakes
- ½ teaspoon dried oregano
- 1 teaspoon dried basil
- 1 ½ cup water
- 1 tablespoon apple cider vinegar
- ¾ cup of coconut milk
- 1 teaspoon nutritional yeast

Directions:

10.   Put in the instant pot: chopped white potato, sweet potato, carrot, and peanuts.

11.   Add water. Close and seal the lid.

12.   Cook the vegetables on manual mode (high pressure) for 6 minutes.

13.   Then allow natural pressure release.

14.   Open the lid. Transfer the contents of the instant pot in the food processor.

15.   Add lime juice, salt, onion powder, ground black pepper, chili flakes, dried oregano, dried basil, apple cider vinegar, coconut milk, and nutritional yeast.

16.   Blend the mixture until smooth and homogenous.

17.   Transfer the cooked cheese sauce in the serving bowl.

Nutrition value/serving: calories 280, fat 19.9, fiber 5.3, carbs 21.9, protein 7.9

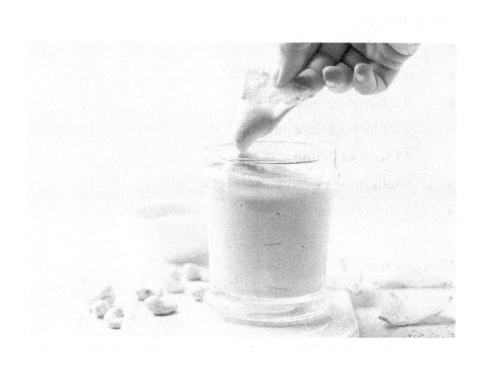

Beetroot Garlic Filling

Prep time: 20 minutes Cooking time: 10 minutes Servings: 4

Ingredients:
- 1 cup beetroot, cubed
- 1 tablespoon garlic, diced
- 1 tablespoon olive oil
- 1 tablespoon lime juice
- ¼ teaspoon lime zest
- 1 tablespoon fresh parsley, chopped
- 1 cup of water

Directions:

14. Put beetroot and water in the instant pot.

15. Close and seal the lid. Cook the vegetables for 10 minutes on Manual mode (high pressure). Then allow natural pressure release for 10 minutes more.

16. Drain water and transfer beetroot in the bowl.

17. Add garlic, lime juice, olive oil, lime zest, and chopped parsley. Stir the filling carefully and let for 10 minutes to marinate.

Nutrition value/serving: calories 53, fat 3.6, fiber 1, carbs 5.3, protein 0.9

Avocado Pesto

Prep time: 10 minutes Cooking time: 5 minutes Servings: 7

Ingredients:
- 2 cups spinach, chopped
- 1 tablespoon olive oil
- 1 teaspoon minced garlic
- 1 tablespoon fresh basil
- 1 tablespoon lemon juice
- 1 avocado, peeled, chopped
- ¼ cup sesame oil
- 1 teaspoon salt
- ½ teaspoon cayenne pepper

Directions:
15. Place chopped spinach and olive oil in the instant pot.
16. Add lemon juice and salt. Stir well.
17. Cook the greens on saute mode for 5 minutes.
18. Transfer the cooked spinach in the blender.
19. Add minced garlic, fresh basil, avocado, sesame oil, and cayenne pepper.

20.   Blend the mixture until smooth.

21.   Pour the cooked pesto sauce in the sauce bowl.

Nutrition value/serving: calories 148, fat 15.5, fiber 2.2, carbs 3, protein 0.9

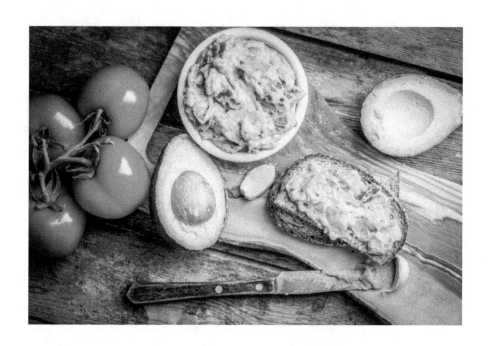

Pear Filling

Prep time: 15 minutes Cooking time: 10 minutes Servings: 4

Ingredients:

- 2 cups pears, chopped
- 1 teaspoon ground cinnamon
- ½ teaspoon ground clove
- 1 tablespoon maple syrup
- 2 tablespoons brown sugar

Directions:

22.   Place pears in the instant pot.

23.   Sprinkle them with ground cinnamon, clove, maple syrup, and brown sugar.

24.   Mix up the fruits well and let them rest for 5-10 minutes or until they start to give juice.

25.   After this, cook filling on Saute mode for 10 minutes. Stir it from time to time.

26.   Chill the filling well.

Nutrition value/serving: calories 79, fat 0.2, fiber 2.9, carbs 20.7, protein 0.3

Mushroom Sauce

Prep time: 5 minutes Cooking time: 4 minutes Servings: 4

Ingredients:

- 1 cup mushrooms, grinded
- 1 onion, grinded
- 1 cup of coconut milk
- 1 teaspoon salt
- 1 teaspoon white pepper
- ¼ teaspoon ground thyme

Directions:

12. Place grinded mushrooms and onion in the instant pot.
13. Add salt, white pepper, and ground thyme.
14. After this, add coconut milk and mix up the mixture well.
15. Close the lid and set manual mode. Cook the sauce for 4 minutes.
16. Then use quick pressure release.
17. Open the lid and mix up the cooked sauce well.

Nutrition value/serving: calories 154, fat 14.4, fiber 2.3, carbs 6.9, protein 2.3

White Bean Sauce

Prep time: 10 minutes Cooking time: 35 minutes Servings: 4

Ingredients:

- ½ cup white beans, soaked
- 1 ½ cup water
- ½ cup almond milk
- 1 tablespoon smoked paprika
- 1 teaspoon salt
- 1 cup fresh parsley, chopped
- 5 oz vegan Parmesan, grated

Directions:

11.	Place white beans, water, almond milk, smoked paprika, salt, and chopped parsley in the instant pot.

12.	Close and seal the lid.

13.	Cook the beans on Manual mode (high pressure) for 35 minutes.

14.	Then use the quick pressure release.

15.	Open the lid and add grated cheese. Mix up the sauce well until cheese is melted.

Nutrition value/serving: calories 272, fat 7.7, fiber 5.7, carbs 26, protein 21.8

Caramel Pumpkin Sauce

Prep time: 5 minutes Cooking time: 3 hours Servings: 6

Ingredients:

- 6 oz pumpkin puree
- 8 oz almond milk
- 1 cup of sugar
- 1 teaspoon ground cinnamon
- 1 teaspoon coconut oil

Directions:

12.   Put all the ingredients in the instant pot and mix up them well.

13.   Close the lid and cook the sauce on Low-pressure mode for 3 hours.

Nutrition value/serving: calories 229, fat 9.9, fiber 1.9, carbs 38, protein 1.2

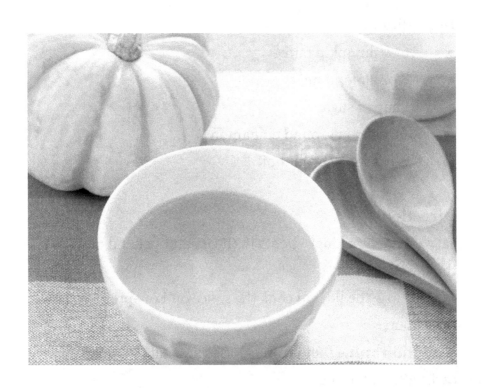

Ravioli Sauce

Prep time: 10 minutes Cooking time: 18 minutes Servings: 5

Ingredients:

- 1 cup tomatoes, canned, chopped
- ½ cup tomato juice
- 2 tablespoons almond yogurt
- 1 teaspoon chili pepper
- 1 teaspoon chili flakes
- 1 teaspoon salt
- ½ teaspoon paprika
- ½ teaspoon ground oregano
- ½ teaspoon ground ginger
- 1 onion, diced
- 1 teaspoon olive oil

Directions:

15.   Preheat instant pot on Saute mode.

16.   Add olive oil and diced onion. Saute it for 3 minutes.

17.   After this, add chopped canned tomatoes, tomato juice, chili pepper, chili flakes, salt, paprika, ground oregano, ground ginger, and stir the sauce well.

18.   Close the lid and cook it on Saute mode for 15 minutes.

19.   Then switch off the instant pot, add almond yogurt, mix it up, and chill the sauce till the room temperature.

Nutrition value/serving: calories 34, fat 1.3, fiber 1.3, carbs 5.4, protein 0.9

Queso Sauce

Prep time: 5 minutes Cooking time: 3 minutes Servings: 4

Ingredients:
- ½ can chilies, chopped, drained
- 6 oz cashew
- ½ teaspoon taco seasoning
- ½ red onion, diced
- 1 teaspoon olive oil
- 1 teaspoon paprika
- ¼ cup of water

Directions:
14. Pour olive oil in the instant pot.
15. Set Saute mode and preheat it.
16. Add red onion and saute it until it is soft.
17. Then transfer the cooked onion in the food processor.
18. Add cashew, chopped chilies, paprika, water, and taco seasoning.
19. Blend the mixture until you get a smooth sauce.
20. Store the sauce in the fridge in the closed container up to 2 days.

Nutrition value/serving: calories 265, fat 21, fiber 1.9, carbs 16.4, protein 6.8

Basil Cream Sauce

Prep time: 10 minutes Cooking time: 2 minutes Servings: 6

Ingredients:

- 1 cup coconut cream
- ½ cup of water
- 1 cup fresh basil, chopped
- 1 garlic clove, peeled
- 1 teaspoon salt
- 1 teaspoon Italian spices
- 1 teaspoon nutritional yeast

Directions:

15. Place fresh basil in the instant pot.

16. Add water and coconut cream.

17. Sprinkle the greens with salt and Italian seasoning.

18. Close and seal the lid.

19. Cook basil for 2 minutes on high-pressure mode. Use quick pressure release.

20. Open the lid and add garlic clove. Blend the mixture until smooth.

21. When the mixture gets to room temperature, add nutritional yeast and mix up well.

22.   Transfer the sauce in the serving bowl.

Nutrition value/serving: calories 96, fat 9.6, fiber 1.1, carbs 2.8, protein 1.3

Creamy Green Peas Filling

Prep time: 10 minutes Cooking time: 5 minutes Servings: 4

Ingredients:

- 2 cups green peas, frozen
- 2 cups of water
- ½ cup coconut cream
- 1 teaspoon tahini paste
- 1 oz fresh dill, chopped

Directions:

17.   Place green peas and water in the instant pot.

18.   Close and seal the lid. Cook green peas for 5 minutes on manual mode.

19.   After this, use quick pressure release.

20.   Open the lid and drain the water.

21.   Then transfer the green peas in the food processor.

22.   Add coconut cream, tahini paste, and chopped dill. Blend it until homogenous.

23.   Store the filling in the closed container in the fridge up to 4 days.

Nutrition value/serving: calories 153, fat 8.4, fiber 5.4, carbs 16.4, protein 6.3

Tomato Sauce

Prep time: 10 minutes Cooking time: 10 minutes Servings: 4

Ingredients:
- 1 tablespoon tomato paste
- 1 cup of water
- 1 tablespoon coconut cream
- 1 tablespoon onion, diced
- 1 teaspoon cornstarch
- 1 teaspoon ground black pepper
- ½ teaspoon chili pepper

Directions:

14. In the instant pot mix up together tomato paste and water.

15. When the mixture changes color to red, add coconut cream, diced onion, ground black pepper, and chili pepper.

16. Close and seal the lid.

17. Cook the sauce for 10 minutes. Use quick pressure release.

18. After this, open the lid and add cornstarch. Stir the sauce until it gets the homogenous texture.

19. Chill it well before serving.

Nutrition value/serving: calories 17, fat 0.9, fiber 0.5, carbs 2.2, protein 0.4

Alfredo Sauce

Prep time: 10 minutes Cooking time: 8 minutes Servings: 4

Ingredients:

- 1 teaspoon minced garlic
- 1 tablespoon avocado oil
- 2 cups cauliflower, chopped
- 3 tablespoons cashews, chopped
- 1 cup of water
- 1 cup of coconut milk
- 1 teaspoon salt

Directions:

14. Pour water and coconut milk in the instant pot.

15. Add chopped cauliflower, salt, and minced garlic.

16. Then add avocado oil. Close and seal the lid.

17. Cook the mixture for 8 minutes on High-pressure mode (manual mode).

18. Then use quick pressure release and open the lid.

19. Add cashews and blend the mixture with the help of the hand blender.

20. When the sauce gets a smooth texture, it is cooked.

Nutrition value/serving: calories 193, fat 17.8, fiber 2.9, carbs 8.5, protein 3.4

Spaghetti Sauce

Prep time: 15 minutes Cooking time: 10 minutes Servings: 2

Ingredients:

- 1 white onion, peeled
- 1 cup tomatoes, chopped
- ½ carrot, chopped
- 1 teaspoon salt
- 1 teaspoon ground black pepper
- 1 garlic clove
- ½ teaspoon sugar
- 1 teaspoon tomato paste

Directions:

15.   Put all the ingredients in the instant pot.

16.   Close and seal the lid. Cook mixture on Manual mode (high pressure) for 10 minutes.

17.   Then allow natural pressure release for 10 minutes.

18.   Open the lid and blend the mixture with the help of the hand blender.

19.   Transfer the cooked sauce in the bowl and chill little.

Nutrition value/serving: calories 55, fat 0.3, fiber 3.1, carbs 12.8, protein 1.9

Marinara Sauce

Prep time: 15 minutes Cooking time: 10 minutes Servings: 4

Ingredients:

- 1 tablespoon onion, minced
- 3 oz bell pepper, chopped
- 1 teaspoon ground black pepper
- ½ teaspoon dried oregano
- ½ teaspoon apple cider vinegar
- ½ cup tomatoes, chopped
- ½ teaspoon tomato paste
- ¼ teaspoon minced garlic
- ¾ cup red wine
- 1/3 teaspoon salt
- ½ teaspoon sugar
- 1 oz mushrooms, chopped
- ¾ cup of water

Directions:

26.   On the saute mode, cook minced onion bell pepper, and tomato paste for 3-4 minutes. Stir it.

27.   Add ground black pepper, dried oregano, apple cider vinegar, chopped tomatoes, minced garlic, red wine, salt, and sugar.

28.   Then add water and mushrooms. Mix up the mixture.

29.   Close and seal the lid.

30.   Cook the sauce on manual mode for 5 minutes. Then allow natural pressure release for 10 minutes.

31.   Chill the sauce well before serving.

Nutrition value/serving: calories 77, fat 0.3, fiber 1.8, carbs 10.5, protein 1.5

Tomato Bean Pate

Prep time: 10 minutes Cooking time: 35 minutes Servings: 4

Ingredients:

- 1 cup red kidney beans, soaked
- 1 teaspoon tomato paste
- 1 teaspoon coconut oil
- 3 cups of water
- 1 teaspoon salt
- 1 carrot, peeled
- 1 teaspoon ground black pepper

Directions:

23.   Place red kidney beans, water, and carrot in the instant pot.

24.   Close and seal the lid.

25.   Cook beans on high-pressure mode for 35 minutes.

26.   Then use quick pressure release.

27.   Open the lid and drain water.

28.   Transfer beans and carrot in the blender.

29.   Add tomato paste, coconut oil, salt, and ground black pepper.

30. Blend the mixture until it gets a soft and smooth texture.

31. Transfer the cooked pate in the bowl.

Nutrition value/serving: calories 173, fat 1.7, fiber 7.6, carbs 30.3, protein 10.6

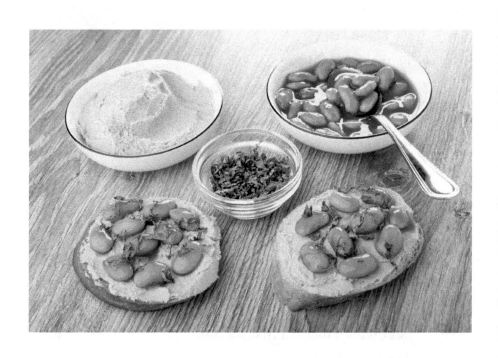

Mint Filling

Prep time: 5 minutes Cooking time: 4 minutes Servings: 2

Ingredients:
- ¼ cup of rice
- 1 cup of water
- 1 teaspoon almond butter
- 1 tablespoon dried mint
- ½ cup corn kernels, frozen
- 1 teaspoon salt

Directions:
23. Place rice and water in the instant pot.
24. Add dried mint and corn kernels. Add salt.
25. Close and seal the lid.
26. Set manual mode and cook filling for 4 minutes. Use quick pressure release.
27. Open the lid and transfer filling in the mixing bowl.
28. Add almond butter and mix up well.

Nutrition value/serving: calories 168, fat 5.1, fiber 2.3, carbs 27.5, protein 4.7

Artichoke Sandwich Filling

Prep time: 10 minutes Cooking time: 15 minutes Servings: 4

Ingredients:
- ½ cup artichoke petals
- 1 cup almond milk
- 3 oz vegan Parmesan, grated
- 1 teaspoon cayenne pepper
- 1 tablespoon cashew butter
- 1 teaspoon olive oil

Directions:
27.   Pour almond milk in the instant pot.

28.   Add artichoke petals, cayenne pepper, cashew butter, and olive oil.

29.   Close the lid and cook the mixture on saute mode for 15 minutes.

30.   When the time is over, add grated cheese and let the mixture stay for 10 minutes more.

31.   Stir the filling well before serving.

Nutrition value/serving: calories 246, fat 17.6, fiber 2.4, carbs 10.6, protein

11.3

Caramel Sauce for Vegetables

Prep time: 10 minutes Cooking time: 2.5 hours Servings: 4

Ingredients:

- ½ cup of sugar
- ½ cup applesauce
- ¾ cup of water
- 1 tablespoon lemon juice
- 1 teaspoon ground coriander

Directions:

21.   Preheat instant pot well.

22.   Add applesauce, water, lemon juice, and ground coriander.

23.   Bring the mixture to boil.

24.   After this, add sugar and stir well.

25.   Close the lid and set low-pressure mode.

26.   Cook the sauce for 2.5 hours.

27.   Chill the cooked sauce well.

Nutrition value/serving: calories 108, fat 0.1, fiber 0.4, carbs 28.5, protein 0.1

Spinach Sauce

Prep time: 10 minutes Cooking time: 6 minutes Servings: 4

Ingredients:

- 1 cup broccoli
- 2 cups spinach, chopped
- 2 cups of water
- 1 teaspoon olive oil
- 1 teaspoon sriracha
- 1 tablespoon lime juice
- 2 oz avocado, chopped
- 1 tablespoon peanuts

Directions:

29.   Chop broccoli and place in the instant pot.

30.   Add water and close the lid.

31.   Cook broccoli on manual mode for 6 minutes. Then use quick pressure release.

32.   Drain ½ part of water.

33.   Place broccoli and remaining water in the food processor.

34.   Add spinach, olive oil, sriracha, lime juice, chopped avocado, and peanuts.

35.   Blend the sauce mixture until smooth.

36.   Transfer the cooked sauce in the glass jar and close the lid. Stor it in the fridge for up to 2 days.

Nutrition value/serving: calories 65, fat 5.2, fiber 2.1, carbs 4.2, protein 1.9

Coconut Filling

Prep time: 5 minutes Cooking time: 3 minutes Servings: 5

Ingredients:
- 1 cup coconut shred
- 1 cup pumpkin puree
- ½ teaspoon ground cardamom
- 1 teaspoon almond butter
- 1 teaspoon sugar

Directions:

27.   Place coconut shred, pumpkin puree, and sugar in the instant pot.

28.   Add almond butter and ground cardamom. Stir it.

29.   Close and seal the lid.

30.   Cook the filling for 3 minutes. Then use quick pressure release.

31.   Chill the filling well.

Nutrition value/serving: calories 133, fat 8.6, fiber 2.6, carbs 14.4, protein 1.8

Ginger Sauce

Prep time: 10 minutes Cooking time: 8 minutes Servings: 4

Ingredients:

- ½ cup of water
- ¾ cup soy sauce
- 1 tablespoon rice vinegar
- 1 teaspoon sesame seeds
- 1 teaspoon minced garlic
- 1 tablespoon minced ginger
- ½ tablespoon sugar
- 1 teaspoon olive oil

Directions:

27.   Preheat instant pot on saute mode well.

28.   Transfer in the instant pot water, soy sauce, rice vinegar, sugar, and olive oil.

29.   Bring the mixture to boil.

30.   After this, pour it in the glass bottle.

31.   Add sesame seeds, minced garlic, and minced ginger. Close the bottle and shake it well.

32.   Leave it for 10 minutes to rest.

Nutrition value/serving: calories 53, fat 1.6, fiber 0.7, carbs 6.5, protein 3.3

Tahini Sauce with Orange Juice

Prep time: 5 minutes Cooking time: 5 minutes Servings: 2

Ingredients:
- 1/3 cup orange juice
- 3 oz tahini
- ½ teaspoon minced garlic
- 1 teaspoon olive oil

Directions:

18. Set saute mode and pour orange juice in the instant pot.
19. Add minced garlic and olive oil.
20. Preheat the mixture until it hot but doesn't start to boil.
21. Transfer the orange juice mixture in the jar.
22. Add tahini and whisk well.
23. Chill it.

Nutrition value/serving: calories 293, fat 25.3, fiber 4, carbs 13.5, protein 7.6

Sriracha Sauce

Prep time: 7 minutes Cooking time: 4 hours Servings: 4

Ingredients:
- 1 cup red chili peppers, chopped
- 1/3 cup water
- ½ cup apple cider vinegar
- 1 teaspoon sugar
- ½ teaspoon salt

Directions:
26. Blend the chili peppers in the blender and transfer the mixture in the instant pot.
27. Add water, apple cider vinegar, sugar, and salt. Mix it up.
28. Close the lid.
29. Cook sauce on low-pressure mode for 4 hours.

Nutrition value/serving: calories 40, fat 0.5, fiber 2.7, carbs 7.7, protein 1

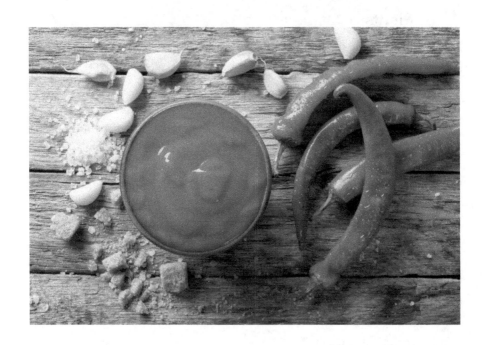

Chimichurri Sauce

Prep time: 15 minutes Cooking time: 11 minutes Servings: 2

Ingredients:
- 2 tablespoons wine vinegar
- 1 oz fresh parsley, chopped
- 1 teaspoon dried oregano
- ½ teaspoon garlic, diced
- ¼ teaspoon chili flakes
- ½ teaspoon ground black pepper
- ¼ cup olive oil

Directions:
26. Pour oil in the instant pot and preheat it on Saute mode.
27. Add dried oregano, chili flakes, and ground black pepper.
28. Stir the mixture and cook it for 1 minute.
29. After this, add wine vinegar and chopped parsley. Stir it well.
30. Switch off the instant pot and let sauce chill till the room temperature.

Nutrition value/serving: calories 231 fat 25.4, fiber 1.9, carbs 21, protein 0.6

Guacamole with Broccoli

Prep time: 10 minutes Cooking time: 2 minutes Servings: 2

Ingredients:

- 1 cup broccoli florets
- ½ cup almond yogurt
- 1 cup of water
- 1 teaspoon salt
- ½ jalapeno, chopped
- ½ red onion, diced
- 2 tablespoons lemon juice
- 1 teaspoon fresh cilantro, chopped
- ¼ cup tomatoes, chopped
- ¼ teaspoon ground black pepper

Directions:

22.   Cook broccoli: put broccoli florets and water in the instant pot.

23.   Close and seal the lid; cook broccoli for 2 minutes on high- pressure mode. Use quick pressure release.

24.   Drain water and transfer broccoli in the blender.

25.   Add salt, chopped jalapeno, almond yogurt, diced onion, lemon juice, cilantro, and ground black pepper.

26.   Blend the mixture well.

27.   Transfer it in the bowl and mix up with the chopped tomatoes.

Nutrition value/serving: calories 116, fat 1.9, fiber 3.8, carbs 23.7, protein 2.5

Miso Butter

Prep time: 10 minutes Cooking time: 7 minutes Servings: 4

Ingredients:
- 1 cups carrot, chopped
- 4 teaspoon tahini paste
- 2 teaspoons maple syrup
- 1 tablespoon miso paste
- 3 tablespoons water
- 1 cup water, for cooking

Directions:
20.   Place carrot and 1 cup of water in the instant pot.

21.   Close and seal the lid.

22.   Cook carrot on high-pressure mode for 7 minutes. Allow natural pressure release for 10 minutes.

23.   Drain the water and transfer hot carrot in the blender.

24.   Add tahini paste, maple syrup, miso paste, and 3 tablespoons of water.

25.   Blend the mixture until you get the smooth buttery texture.

26.   Transfer it in the bowl for butter.

Nutrition value/serving: calories 58, fat 3, fiber 1.4, carbs 7.1, protein 1.6

Vegan Buffalo Dip

Prep time: 10 minutes Cooking time: 4 minutes Servings: 3

Ingredients:

- 1 cup cauliflower, chopped
- 1 cup of water
- ½ cup chickpeas, canned
- 1/3 cup almond milk
- 1 teaspoon salt
- 4 teaspoons hot sauce
- 1 tablespoon lemon juice
- 1 teaspoon garlic powder

Directions:

23. Place cauliflower and water in the instant pot.

24. Close and seal the lid; cook the vegetable for 4 minutes on manual mode.

25. Then use quick pressure release.

26. Open the lid and drain water.

27. Transfer cauliflower in the blender.

28. Add chickpeas, almond milk, salt, hot sauce, lemon juice, and garlic powder.

29. Blend it until smooth.

30.   Transfer cooked Buffalo dip in the serving bowl.

Nutrition value/serving: calories 196, fat 8.5, fiber 7.4, carbs 24.4, protein 7.9

Oregano Onion Dip

Prep time: 10 minutes Cooking time: 10 minutes Servings: 5

Ingredients:
- 3 cups onions, chopped
- 2 cups of coconut milk
- 1 teaspoon coconut butter
- 1 teaspoon salt
- 1 teaspoon white pepper
- 1 teaspoon paprika
- 1 teaspoon wheat flour
- 1 tablespoon dried oregano

Directions:
28.   Toss coconut butter in the instant pot and melt it on Saute mode.

29.   Add chopped onions and sprinkle them with salt, white pepper, paprika, and dried oregano.

30.   Stir well and cook on saute mode for 5 minutes.

31.   After this, add wheat flour and coconut milk. Mix up the mixture.

32.   Close and seal the lid.

33.   Cook the onion dip on manual mode for 4 minutes. Then allow natural pressure release for 5 minutes more.

34.   Chill the cooked meal to room temperature.

Nutrition value/serving: calories 262, fat 23.7, fiber 4.4, carbs 13.5, protein 3.3

Baba Ganoush

Prep time: 10 minutes Cooking time: 10 minutes Servings: 8

Ingredients:

- 2 eggplants
- ¼ cup fresh cilantro, chopped
- ¾ cup lime juice
- ½ teaspoon garlic, diced
- 4 teaspoons tahini
- ½ teaspoon salt
- 1 cup water, for cooking

Directions:

31. Pour water in the instant pot. Insert rack.

32. Peel the eggplants and place them on the rack.

33. Close the lid and cook vegetables on Steam mode for 10 minutes.

34. When the time is over, transfer the eggplants in the blender.

35. Add lime juice, garlic, tahini, and salt.

36. Blend the mixture until smooth.

37. Add fresh cilantro and pulse the mixture for 5 seconds more.

---

38.   Transfer the cooked meal in the serving bowl.

Nutrition value/serving: calories 56, fat 1.7, fiber 5.2, carbs 10.7, protein 1.9

Chili Sauce

Prep time: 8 minutes Cooking time: 8 minutes Servings: 4

Ingredients:

- 2 chili peppers
- 1 cup tomatoes
- ½ teaspoon tomato paste
- ¼ cup of water
- 1 teaspoon diced garlic
- 1 date, chopped
- 1 tablespoon rice vinegar
- 1 cup water, for cooking

Directions:

24. Pour 1 cup of water in the instant pot and insert rack.

25. Place chili peppers and tomatoes on the rack.

26. Close and seal the lid.

27. Cook the vegetables on Steam mode for 8 minutes.

28. Transfer the cooked peppers and tomatoes in the blender.

29. Add tomato paste, ¼ cup water, diced garlic, chopped date, and rice vinegar.

30. Blend the sauce until it reaches the desired structure.

Nutrition value/serving: calories 19, fat 0.1, fiber 0.8, carbs 3.8, protein 0.6

Walnut Sauce

Prep time: 7 minutes Cooking time: 4 minutes Servings: 2

Ingredients:

- 1/3 cup walnuts, chopped
- 1 white onion, peeled
- ½ teaspoon minced garlic
- 1 tablespoon olive oil
- 1 teaspoon ground black pepper
- ½ teaspoon salt
- ½ cup water, for cooking

Directions:

29.   Place onion and water in the instant pot.

30.   Close and seal the lid. Cook onion for 4 minutes on Manual mode. Use quick pressure release.

31.   Drain water from the instant pot and transfer the onion in the blender.

32.   Add walnuts, minced garlic, olive oil, ground black pepper, and salt.

33.   Blend the sauce well.

Nutrition value/serving: calories 214, fat 19.4, fiber 2.9, carbs 8.1, protein 5.8

Green Goddess Sauce

Prep time: 10 minutes Cooking time: 2 minutes Servings: 4

Ingredients:

- 6 oz avocado, mashed
- 2 cups spinach, chopped
- 1 teaspoon wine vinegar
- 1 tablespoon lemon juice
- 1 cup fresh parsley, chopped
- 3 oz scallions, chopped
- ½ garlic clove, diced
- 1 teaspoon salt
- 1 teaspoon chili pepper
- ½ cup water, for cooking

Directions:

28.   In the instant pot combine together ½ cup of water and spinach.

29.   Close and seal the lid. Cook spinach for 2 minutes. Use quick pressure release.

30.   After this, transfer the water and spinach in the blender.

31. Add avocado mash, wine vinegar, lemon juice, chopped parsley, scallions, garlic clove, salt, and chili pepper.

32. Blend the mixture until smooth.

33. Stir the sauce in the closed glass jar up to 2 days.

Nutrition value/serving: calories 106, fat 8.6, fiber 4.6, carbs 11.8, protein 2.2

Herbed Lemon Sauce

Prep time: 5 minutes Cooking time: 5 minutes Servings: 3

Ingredients:
- 1 teaspoon lemon juice
- 1 tablespoon almond butter
- 1 teaspoon cornstarch
- ½ cup of water
- 2 teaspoons sugar
- ½ teaspoon salt
- ¼ teaspoon lemon zest

Directions:
27.   Pour water in the instant pot and preheat it on Saute mode.

28.   Add cornstarch and stir carefully until homogenous.

29.   After this, add lemon juice, almond butter, sugar, salt, and lemon zest.

30.   Whisk the mixture well and bring it to boil.

31.   Then switch off the instant pot and chill the sauce.

Nutrition value/serving: calories 47, fat 3, fiber 0.6, carbs 4.6, protein 1.1

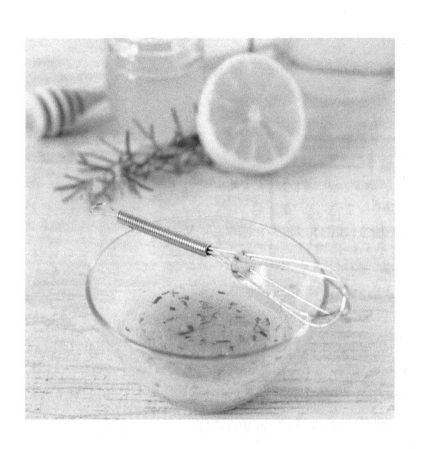

Roasted Pepper Salsa

Prep time: 10 minutes Cooking time: 5 minutes Servings: 4

Ingredients:
- 1-pound sweet pepper, seeded
- 1 cup tomatoes, chopped
- 1 oz fresh basil
- 1 teaspoon salt
- 1 teaspoon ground black pepper
- 1 garlic clove, chopped
- 1 tablespoon balsamic vinegar
- 2 tablespoons olive oil
- 1 cup water, for cooking

Directions:
28. Pour water in the instant pot. Insert the trivet.

29. Place sweet peppers on the trivet and close the lid.

30. Cook them on Manual mode (high pressure) for 5 minutes.

31. Then use quick pressure release.

32. Open the lid and transfer the peppers in the blender.

33. Add tomatoes, fresh basil, salt, ground black pepper, garlic, balsamic vinegar, and olive oil.

34. Blend the mixture for 1 minute.

35. Transfer the cooked salsa in the serving bowl.

Nutrition value/serving: calories 82, fat 7.2, fiber 1.2, carbs 4.8, protein 1

Arugula Hummus

Prep time: 25 minutes Cooking time: 25 minutes Servings: 4

Ingredients:

- 1 cup garbanzo beans, soaked
- 3 cups of water
- 2 cups arugula
- 1 teaspoon salt
- 1 teaspoon harissa
- 1 tablespoon olive oil
- 1 teaspoon lemon juice
- ½ teaspoon tahini

Directions:

29. Cook garbanzo beans: place water and beans in the instant pot.

30. Close and seal the lid; cook the beans for 25 minutes, then allow natural pressure release for 20 minutes more.

31. After this, transfer beans and 1/3 cup of bean water in the blender.

32. Add arugula, salt, harissa, olive oil, lemon juice, and tahini.

33. Blend the mixture until smooth.

34.   Transfer arugula hummus in the serving bowl.

Nutrition value/serving: calories 223, fat 7.2, fiber 8.9, carbs 31.4, protein 10.1

Edamole

Prep time: 10 minutes Cooking time: 8 minutes Servings: 4

Ingredients:

- 1 cup green soybeans, soaked
- 4 cups of water
- 1 garlic clove, chopped
- ½ teaspoon ground cumin
- 1 tablespoon hot sauce

Directions:

25. Place water and soybeans in the instant pot.

26. Close and seal the lid.

27. Cook soybeans on manual mode for 30 minutes. Then use quick pressure release.

28. Drain water and transfer soybeans in the blender.

29. Add garlic clove, ground cumin, and hot sauce.

30. Blend the mixture for 1-2 minutes.

31. Transfer edamole in the serving bowl.

Nutrition value/serving: calories 210, fat 9.3, fiber 4.4, carbs 14.5, protein 17.1

Pizza Sauce

Prep time: 5 minutes Cooking time: 6 minutes Servings: 6

Ingredients:

- ½ cup tomato juice
- ¼ cup almond yogurt
- 1 teaspoon minced garlic
- 1 teaspoon dried dill
- 1 teaspoon Italian seasoning
- 1 teaspoon maple syrup
- 1 teaspoon chili pepper
- 1 teaspoon olive oil

Directions:

23.   Pour olive oil in the instant pot. Preheat it on Saute mode.

24.   Add chili pepper, Italian seasoning, dried dill, and minced garlic.

25.   Cook the mixture for 2 minutes. Stir it.

26.   Then add maple syrup, tomato juice, and almond yogurt. Mix up the mixture.

27.   Close the lid and saute sauce for 4 minutes.

28.   Then open the lid, mix up the sauce one more time and transfer it in the bowl.

Nutrition value/serving: calories 24, fat 1.4, fiber 0.2, carbs 2.8, protein 0.4

Garlic Dip

Prep time: 15 minutes Cooking time: 5 minutes Servings: 2

Ingredients:

- ½ cup almond milk
- ¼ cup garlic, minced
- 1 teaspoon salt
- ½ teaspoon ground black pepper
- 1 teaspoon cornflour

Directions:

31.   Pour almond milk in the instant pot.

32.   Preheat it on Saute mode.

33.   Add cornflour and whisk well.

34.   Then add minced garlic, salt, and ground black pepper.

35.   Keep whisking dip for 3 minutes more.

36.   Then switch off the instant pot and close the lid.

37.   Let the dip rest for 10-15 minutes before serving.

Nutrition value/serving: calories 169, fat 14.5, fiber 1.9, carbs 10.2, protein 2.6

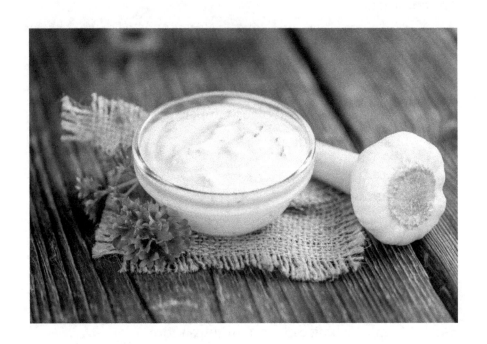

CPSIA information can be obtained
at www.ICGtesting.com
Printed in the USA
LVHW021316060521
686680LV00017B/1116